Skinny
HALOGEN
OVEN COOKING FOR ONE

CookNation

Skinny Halogen Oven Cooking For One
Single Serving, Healthy, Low Calorie Halogen Oven
Recipes Under 200, 300 and 400 Calories

A Bell & Mackenzie Publication
First published in 2013 by Bell & Mackenzie Publishing
Copyright © Bell & Mackenzie Publishing 2013

ISBN 978-1-909855-04-5

Disclaimer
The information and advice in this book is intended as
a guide only. Any individual should independently seek
the advice of a health professional before embarking
on a diet. Some recipes may contain nuts or traces of
nuts. Those suffering from any allergies associated with
nuts should avoid any recipes containing nuts or nut
based oils.

Contents

Contents

Contents

Contents

Skinny HALOGEN
OVEN COOKING FOR ONE

INTRODUCTION

Introduction

The halogen oven is a remarkable appliance providing a space saving, economical and affordable way to cook. Cooking for one can sometimes feel uninspiring and if you are also cooking low calorie meals, either to maintain your current weight or as part of a calorie controlled diet, finding healthy calorie friendly single servings can be difficult.

'Skinny Halogen Cooking For One' sets out over 75 delicious, low calorie, homemade meals prepared in your halogen oven. Each recipe is simple to follow, balanced, serves one and all fall below either 200, 300 or 400 calories each. By calculating the number of calories for each dish we've made it easy for you to count your daily calorie intake and cooking times are all under 60 minutes with minimal preparation.

Cooking skinny low calorie meals using your halogen oven couldn't be a simpler way to follow a healthy eating plan. We hope you enjoy all the recipes in this book.

You may also be interested in other CookNation titles in the 'skinny' series listed at the end of this book.

What This Book Will Do For You

The recipes in this book are all low calorie dishes for one which make it easy for you to control your overall daily calorie intake. The recommended daily calories are approximately 2000 for women and 2500 for men. Broadly speaking, by consuming this level of calories each day you should maintain your current weight.

Reducing the number of calories (a calorie deficit) will result in losing weight. This happens because the body begins to use fat stores for energy to make up the reduction in calories, which in turn results in weight loss. We have already counted the calories for each dish making it easy for you to fit this into to your daily eating plan whether you want to lose weight, maintain your current figure or are just looking for some great-tasting easy to prepare halogen oven recipes.

I'm Already On A Diet. Can I Use These Recipes?

Yes of course. All the recipes can be great accompaniments to many popular calorie-counting diets. We all know that sometimes dieting can result in hunger pangs, cravings and boredom from eating the same old foods day in and day out. 'Skinny Halogen Oven Cooking' can break that cycle by providing filling meals for one which satisfy you for hours afterwards.

What is A Halogen Oven?

You may already have a halogen oven or perhaps are contemplating buying one. Either way a brief explanation of this remarkable appliance is worth a little time.

A halogen oven is an electrical countertop appliance which performs the same functions as a traditional oven but can be operated at a fraction of the running cost and results in reduced cooking times.

It uses a powerful halogen bulb, housed in the lid of the unit, to produce radiant infrared heat which, when circulated around the glass bowl of the appliance using a powerful fan, cooks the food evenly and quicker than a traditional fan assisted/gas oven.

Halogen ovens should not be confused with microwave ovens which use radio waves to penetrate food, causing friction between water and fat molecules. This friction provides heat which in turn cooks the food. Typically a halogen oven can reduce cooking times compared to a conventional oven by 20-30% and sometimes by up to 40%. It is worth mentioning that you should be wary of claims that a halogen oven will cut your cooking times in half. If this is your main reason for buying one you may find yourself disappointed with the results.

Every unit will normally come with a low and high grill rack, tongs, a rack to place the lid of the appliance when adding/removing food (it becomes very hot) and sometimes an extender ring to increase the capacity of the oven (these can also be purchased separately). For advice on which model best suits your needs, refer to the *Which Halogen Oven* section later in this book.

What Are The Benefits of Cooking With A Halogen Oven?

Cooking times can be reduced by 20-30% compared to a conventional oven but there are many other advantages to cooking halogen style.

Affordable. Depending which model you choose (more on that later) prices range between $40-$100 or £30-£80. This is a fraction of the cost of a conventional oven .

Economical. As well as the affordable price, halogen ovens are less expensive to run than a conventional oven. Because they are smaller, provide a constant temperature due to the circulation of air and the intense heat of the bulb together with accurate temperature sensors, food cooks in less time, which in turn means less electricity. In addition they heat up very quickly so lengthy pre-heating is generally not needed. However it is worth switching the oven on when you begin recipe preparation so that the oven is ready to go.

Multifunctional. Halogens Ovens have many uses. They can roast, grill, bake, steam, defrost and can even make toast and boiled eggs.

Healthy. Halogen ovens work best by circulating heat around the food. The use of the wire racks that are provided with the unit mean that if you are looking for a healthier way to cook your food, any excess fat produced while cooking drains away. Also, cooking with a halogen oven requires less additional oil and fats.

Visible. One of the great advantages of a halogen oven is you can literally see your food cooking. The large glass bowl enables you to check on your food without opening the appliance as you would in a conventional oven.

Self-cleaning. Although you can remove the glass bowl, most halogen ovens will come with a self-cleaning function. This is a pre-programmed function to clean your bowl using water and dish soap/washing up liquid.

Is There Anything My Halogen Oven Can't Do?

Due to their size, there are limitations on the quantity of food you can cook. If you have a dinner party of 10 then perhaps the help of a conventional oven would be advised. Most appliances will comfortably cater for 4-6 but, for the purposes of this book all recipes are for one serving.

Halogen ovens work best by circulating air around the food so if too much is packed into the bowl, cooking times will increase. Similarly heavily liquid based dishes such as soups will require longer cooking times than you might expect. Vegetables, particularly root vegetables, can take longer than meat to cook in a halogen oven. Pasta and rice should generally be pre-cooked. Tinned pulses and beans are generally better than dried.

All of the above have been taken into consideration in our recipes so don't worry.

Which Halogen Oven?

As with any new purchase you should consider how you will use your appliance and of course the budget you can afford. If you are buying a halogen oven for the first time or replacing a model, we strongly recommend you spend some time researching customer reviews before parting with your money. There are a number of websites dedicated to halogen ovens which provide very useful comparisons. Amazon's customer reviews are also an excellent resource.

Size. Generally halogen ovens come in 7 litre up to 17 litre capacities. 12 litres are generally the most popular. Normally we would advise opting for larger capacity model if your budget can stretch as this will allow you to cook for more people if needed. However as all our recipes serve one, a smaller capacity machine is fine.

Lid: The lid of a halogen cooker is what houses the cooking element. It can be quite heavy and the element is extremely hot when the lid is lifted off after cooking. Most models should come with a lid rack which enables you to place the lid on your counter top (otherwise the element would burn the work surface). If your budget can stretch, buying a model that has a hinged lid is easier and safer as it does not detach from the appliance.

Extras. It is worth researching which manufacturers will offer some handy extras. As standard you should get a low and high rack with your appliance but some also offer, tongs, extender rings, recipe books and replacement bulbs. Always check how long a guarantee is provided with each model.

Tips

* If your model has an extender ring, consider using it so that the element is further away from your food. For dishes that could potentially splash while cooking, this prevents the element from becoming dirty. The element can be difficult to clean so this will keep things manageable. Always wipe down the element when cooled with a damp cloth after cooking.

* Make sure you have enough space on your counter top. Although halogen ovens are relatively compact if you do not own the model with a hinged lid you will have to allow space to remove the lid onto the lid stand.

* Use foil to prevent food from browning too quickly. This is not always necessary but can be a good way to prevent food from burning. Alternatively the extender ring can serve the same purpose by placing the element further from the food.

* Be prepared to adjust cooking times. Groceries are rarely uniform in size and each model of halogen may be slightly different, so increasing or decreasing your oven temperatures and cooking times may be needed.

* Consider which rack to use – low or high. If you need your food to brown the high rack will be best but if you require longer cooking times use the low rack. All our recipes specify which should be used.

* Lay some tin foil on the base of your bowl to catch any cooking juices. This will make washing up much easier.

* Always read the manufactures instructions. These will offer some additional tips and safety guidelines to get the most out of your particular appliance.

All Recipes Are A Guide Only

All the recipes in this book are a guide only. You may need to alter quantities and cooking times to suit your own appliance .

Skinny HALOGEN OVEN
CHICKEN & POULTRY DISHES

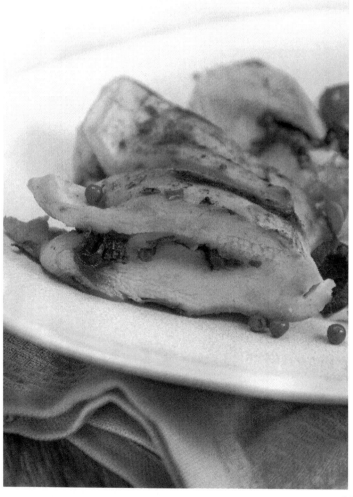

Lemon & Thyme Chicken
Serves 1

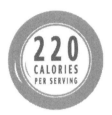

220 CALORIES PER SERVING

Ingredients:

125g/4oz skinless chicken breast
1 garlic clove, crushed
1 tsp freshly chopped thyme leaves

1 lemon
Pinch crushed chilli flakes
50g/2oz rocket leaves
15g/ ½oz parmesan shavings
Salt & pepper to taste

Method:

Chop half of the lemon into slices, squeeze and reserve the juice from the other half. Combine the lemon juice, garlic, thyme and chilli flakes together to create a marinade. Place the chicken breast in an oven proof dish and score the flesh with a knife. Brush the breast with all the marinade, season well and leave for up to 1 hour to marinate.

Carefully cover the chicken breast with the sliced lemon pieces, place on the lower rack and leave to cook in the halogen oven for 25-30 minutes at 200C/400F or until the chicken is cooked through.

Remove the cooked chicken to a plate and serve with the rocket salad and parmesan shavings.

If there is any marinade left in the bowl after cooking, spoon it onto the salad as a dressing. This dish is also good with chopped fresh tomatoes tossed through the rocket leaves.

West Indian Coconut Chicken With Rice & Plantain

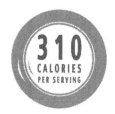

Serves 1

Ingredients:

Low-cal cooking oil spray
1 onion, chopped
125g/4oz skinless chicken breast
75g/3oz plantain, peeled & sliced
1 tsp plain/all-purpose flour
½ tsp each cayenne pepper, paprika & mustard seeds

1 tsp freshly grated ginger
1 garlic clove, crushed
Pinch ground cinnamon
60ml/¼ cup hot chicken stock
120ml/½ cup low fat coconut milk
50g long grain rice
Salt & pepper to taste

Method:

Gently sauté the onion, garlic, dried spices and mustard seeds in a little low-cal spray for a few minutes until the onion softens and the mustard seeds begin to pop. Stir through the flour and add the hot chicken stock to the pan. Continue stirring for a minute or two. Combine all the ingredients, except the coconut milk in an ovenproof dish. Place on the lower rack and leave to cook in the halogen oven at 180C/350F for 30-35 minutes or until the chicken is cooked through and the plantain is tender. Meanwhile cook the rice in salted boiling water until tender. When the chicken is cooked gently stir through the coconut milk, season and serve with the boiled rice.

Plantain is a starchy type of banana which must be cooked before eating and is used widely in Caribbean cooking. They are readily available in the UK & US, however feel free to substitute sweet potatoes in this recipe if you prefer.

Red Onion & Green Pesto Chicken

Serves 1

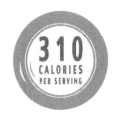

310 CALORIES PER SERVING

Ingredients:

Low-cal cooking oil spray
125g/4oz skinless chicken breast
½ onion, sliced
1 tsp green pesto

1 tsp dried oregano
1 red onion, sliced into rounds
50g/2oz French beans
50g/2oz baby corn
Salt & pepper to taste

Method:

Hold the chicken breast as if you were slicing through the centre of it to butterfly it. Stop slicing before you cut it in half completely. Open the chicken breast to expose the two inside parts. Spread the inside with the pesto and close your 'sandwich' back up so you are left with pesto through the centre of the chicken breast. Place the chicken, onions and vegetables in a casserole dish. Season well, sprinkle with the dried oregano and spray with a little low-cal cooking oil.

Place on the lower rack and leave to cook in the halogen oven at 200C/400F for 25-30 minutes or until the chicken is cooked through and the vegetables are tender. Remove from the halogen oven and arrange the beans, corn and onions as a bed onto which you serve the pesto chicken breast.

You could easily make your own pesto for this recipe by pulsing together fresh basil, olive oil, salt, pine nuts, garlic & a little lemon juice.

Creamy Mustard Chicken & New Potatoes

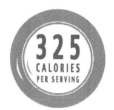

Serves 1

Ingredients:

Low-cal cooking oil spray
125g/4oz skinless chicken breast
1 onion, chopped
50g/2oz chestnut mushrooms, sliced
60ml/¼ cup chicken stock
2 tsp dijon mustard

Splash white wine
3 tbsp low fat crème fraiche
50g/2oz small new potatoes/ halved
50g/2oz spinach leaves
1 tbsp freshly chopped flat leaf parsley
Salt & pepper to taste

Method:

Slice the chicken into strips. Gently sauté the onion and mushrooms in a little low-cal oil for a few minutes. Add the chicken stock and mustard to the pan with a splash of wine and bring to the boil. Continue stirring for a minute or two while it bubbles away. Combine all the ingredients, except the crème fraiche and chopped parsley, in an ovenproof dish. Place on the lower rack and leave to cook in the halogen oven at 180C/350F for 20-25 minutes or until the chicken is cooked through and the potatoes are tender. After cooking gently stir through the crème fraiche, season and serve with the chopped parsley sprinkled over the top.

You could introduce a variety of mustards into this recipe. English mustard will give it a 'hotter' taste whilst wholegrain mustard will give it a little 'depth'.

Spanish Chicken
Serves 1

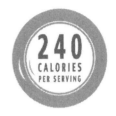

240 CALORIES PER SERVING

Ingredients:

Low-cal cooking oil spray
125g/4oz skinless chicken breast, sliced
1 onion, chopped
1 tsp smoked paprika & dried sage
1 tsp each freshly chopped rosemary & basil leaves
200g/7oz chopped tomatoes

1 yellow (bell) pepper, sliced
75g/3oz uncooked chorizo sausage, sliced
2 garlic cloves, crushed
8 pitted olives, halved
50g/2oz tender stem broccoli, roughly chopped
Salt & pepper to taste

Method:

Gently sauté the onion, sliced pepper, garlic & paprika in a little low-cal oil for a few minutes until softened. Add the sliced chorizo & chicken and cook for 3-4 minutes longer. Combine all the ingredients, except the fresh chopped herbs in a casserole dish. Place on the lower rack and leave to cook in the halogen oven at 200C/400F for 25-30 minutes or until the chicken is cooked through and the vegetables are tender. Season well and serve.

As an alternative try shredding the chicken after cooking and serve warm or cold on low-cal crisp bread or toasted ciabatta slices.

Chicken & Serrano Ham
Serves 1

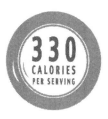

330 CALORIES PER SERVING

Ingredients:

125g/4oz skinless chicken breast
1 tbsp low fat cream cheese with chives
1 slice Serrano ham

3 ripe tomatoes, halved
75g/3oz spinach or spring greens
1 tsp garlic oil
Salt & pepper to taste

Method:

Make a lengthways slit in the chicken breast and stuff with the cream cheese. Season the chicken breast and wrap with the Serrano ham (secure in place with a cocktail stick skewered through the breast). Place in a casserole dish on the lower rack and leave to cook in the halogen oven at 200C/400F for 25-30 minutes or until the chicken is cooked through. Meanwhile mix together the halved tomatoes, garlic oil and spinach leaves so that they all have a thin coating of oil on them. Season well and place around the chicken in the casserole dish 10 minutes before the end of cooking time. Serve in a shallow bowl with the vegetables arranged around the chicken.

You could use any type of thin cured meat to wrap the chicken breast in, or whichever soft cheese and herb variety you prefer.

Boursin & Sundried Tomato Chicken
Serves 1

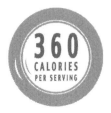

360 CALORIES PER SERVING

Ingredients:

125g/4oz skinless chicken breast
1 tsp Boursin soft cheese
1 tsp sundried tomato paste

½ tsp anchovy paste
75g/3oz steamed broccoli florets
Salt & pepper to taste

Method:

First mix together the Boursin cheese and anchovy paste. Hold the chicken breast as if you were slicing through the centre of it to butterfly it. Stop slicing before you cut it in half completely and open the chicken breast to expose the two inside parts. Spread the inside of the chicken breast with the anchovy & cheese mix and close your 'sandwich' breast back up. Spread the top of the chicken with the sundried tomato paste and cover with foil. Place in an ovenproof dish on the lower rack and leave to cook in the halogen oven at 200C/400F for 25-30 minutes or until the chicken is cooked through. Meanwhile steam the broccoli florets over a pan of boiling water for 5-10 minutes or until tender. Season well and serve with the chicken breast.

Boursin cheese is a lovely flavoursome soft cheese but you may wish to use a lower fat alternative such as Philadelphia cheese if you want to reduce the calories further. Also don't worry if you don't have any anchovy paste, just double the tomato paste.

Almond & Walnut Chicken

Serves 1

390 CALORIES PER SERVING

Ingredients:

125g/4oz skinless chicken breast
½ tsp ground almonds
15g/½oz walnuts, finely chopped
50g/2oz chestnut mushrooms, chopped
½ onion, finely chopped
1 tsp garlic paste
75g/3oz steamed new potatoes
Salt & pepper to taste

Method:

First mix together the ground almonds, walnuts, mushrooms, onion & garlic paste. Make a lengthways slit in the chicken breast and stuff with the walnut mixture. Don't worry if it's overflowing a little, just gently cover in foil to keep it together. Place in an ovenproof dish on the lower rack and leave to cook in the halogen oven at 200C/400F for 25-30 minutes or until the chicken is cooked through. Meanwhile steam the new potatoes over a pan of boiling water for 10-20 minutes or until tender. Season well and serve with the chicken breast.

A crispy crunchy onion salad served on the side is a lovely addition to this meal.

Chicken Tikka Kebabs
Serves 1

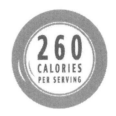

260 CALORIES PER SERVING

Ingredients:

125g/4oz skinless chicken breast, cubed
1 tbsp fat free Greek yoghurt
1 tsp each ground cumin, turmeric, coriander/cilantro & mild chilli powder

1 garlic clove, crushed
2 metal skewers
1 romaine lettuce, shredded
½ red onion, sliced
½ lemon cut into wedges
Salt & pepper to taste

Method:

Season the cubed chicken. Mix together the spices, garlic and yoghurt and add the chicken. Combine well, cover and leave to chill for an hour or two.

Skewer the chicken pieces to make 2 chicken kebabs and place on the grill pan at the top of the halogen oven on 240C/475F. Grill for 6-8 minutes each side or until the chicken is cooked through (take care handling the skewers as they will get hot). Serve with the shredded lettuce, sliced onions and lemon wedges.

If you don't have time to leave the chicken to marinate don't let that put you off making this dish. It will still taste great.

Chicken & Cannellini Beans

Serves 1

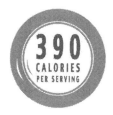

390 CALORIES PER SERVING

Ingredients:

Low-cal cooking oil spray
125g/4oz skinless chicken breast, sliced diagonally
½ onion, chopped
1 tsp each dried oregano, basil & rosemary
200g/7oz tinned chopped tomatoes

200g/7oz tinned cannellini beans, drained
½ yellow (bell) pepper, sliced
1 garlic clove, crushed
1 tbsp worcestershire sauce
1 tbsp tomato puree/paste
Salt & pepper to taste

Method:

Gently sauté the onion, sliced pepper, garlic & herbs in a little low-cal oil for a few minutes until softened. Add the chopped tomatoes and sliced chicken and cook for 3-4 minutes longer. Combine all the ingredients in an ovenproof dish. Place on the lower rack and leave to cook in the halogen oven at 200C/400F for 25-30 minutes or until the chicken is cooked through and the vegetables are tender. Season well and serve.

This is a great simple store cupboard one-pot meal. Any type of dried herbs will do well in this recipe so don't worry if you don't have the exact listed ingredients

Lean Turkey Burger
Serves 1

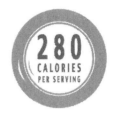

280 CALORIES PER SERVING

Ingredients:

Low-cal cooking oil spray
125g/4oz lean turkey mince
½ piece brown bread
1 egg yolk
½ onion
1 ripe tomato, sliced

1 garlic clove
1 tsp fat free mayonnaise
1 handful shredded lettuce
1 wholemeal brown roll
Salt & pepper to taste

Method:

Place the bread and garlic in a food processor and pulse to make bread crumbs. Add the onion and whizz again. Add the turkey mince and egg yolk and pulse for a few seconds longer until combined. Season well and form into a large burger patty. Spray with a little low cal-cooking oil and place on the grill pan at the top of the halogen oven on 240C/475F. Grill for 5-7 mins each side, or until the burger is cooked through. Spread the mayonnaise on the split burger bun and serve with tomato and lettuce on top.

This burger is a meal in itself. It's worth investing in a plastic burger maker to make perfect burgers shapes. They cost very little and really improve the shape and texture of the patty.

Tandoori Chicken With Mint Yoghurt

Serves 1

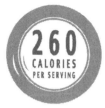

260 CALORIES PER SERVING

Ingredients:

Low-cal cooking oil spray
125g/4oz skinless chicken
breast
1 tsp each ground cumin,
turmeric, coriander/cilantro &
chilli powder
½ tsp each ground ginger &
garam masala

1 tbsp lemon juice
2 garlic cloves, crushed
1 baby gem lettuce, shredded
½ red onion, sliced
½ lemon cut into wedges
2 tbsp fat free Greek yoghurt
1 tsp mint sauce
Salt & pepper to taste

Method:

Mix together the lemon juice, ground spices & garlic to form a
paste (add a little water if needed). Season the chicken breast and
spray with a little low-cal oil. Score the chicken breast all over with
a knife and smother in the spice paste. Place in an ovenproof dish
and leave for up to 1 hour to marinate.

Place on the lower rack and leave to cook in the halogen oven
for 25-30 minutes at 200C/400F or until the chicken is cooked
through. Meanwhile mix the mint sauce and Greek yoghurt
together. Plate up the tandoori chicken breast with the lettuce &
onion and serve the lemon wedges and mint yoghurt on the side.

*Combining shop-bought mint sauce with yoghurt is
a really quick way to make a tasty Indian condiment
which will compliment any spicy dish.*

Honey Roast Chicken & Vegetables
Serves 1

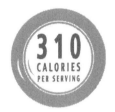

310 CALORIES PER SERVING

Ingredients:

Low-cal cooking oil spray
125g/4oz skinless chicken breast
75g/3oz sweet potatoes, cubed
1 parsnip, cubed
1 carrot, cubed
½ onion chopped

2 vine ripened tomatoes, halved
1 garlic clove, crushed
1 tbsp lemon juice
1 tsp soy sauce
2 tsp runny honey
Salt & pepper to taste

Method:

Mix together the garlic, lemon juice, honey and soy sauce. Brush the chicken and tomatoes with the honey mixture and use the rest to coat the vegetables well in an ovenproof dish. Season and spray with a little low-cal oil. Place on the lower rack and leave to cook for 25-30 minutes or until the chicken is cooked through and the vegetables are tender. 10 minutes before the end of cooking add the tomatoes. Season well and serve.

Any combination of root vegetables works well with this dish, however root vegetables generally take longer to cook than meat so make sure they are tender before serving. You may need to leave the chicken to rest while while the vegetables finish in the oven.

Butter Beans & Fennel Chicken
Serves 1

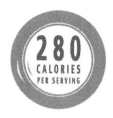

280 CALORIES PER SERVING

Ingredients:

Low-cal cooking oil spray
125g/4oz skinless chicken breast
1 leek, chopped
½ fennel bulb, chopped
200g/7oz tinned butter beans, drained

1 tbsp freshly chopped parsley
120ml/½ cup chicken stock
2 garlic cloves, crushed
75g/3oz tender stem broccoli, roughly chopped
Salt & pepper to taste

Method:

Gently sauté the garlic, leek & fennel in a little low-cal spray for a few minutes until softened. Combine all the ingredients, except the parsley in an ovenproof dish. Place on the lower rack and leave to cook in the halogen oven at 200C/400F for 25-30 minutes or until the chicken is cooked through and the vegetables are tender. Season well and serve with the chopped parsley sprinkled over the top.

Depending on your oven there may be a little liquid left in the casserole dish. This is lovely spooned over the top of the chicken and beans.

Aromatic Chicken
Serves 1

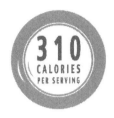

310 CALORIES PER SERVING

Ingredients:

125g/4oz skinless chicken breast
½ tsp each ground paprika, cinnamon, cumin & coriander/cilantro

Pinch nutmeg
2 garlic cloves, crushed
50g/2oz basmati rice
50g/2oz peas
Salt & pepper to taste

Method:

Mix the ground spices and garlic together with a little water to form a paste. Score the chicken breast with a knife and smother in the spice paste. Place on the lower rack, cover with foil and leave to cook in the halogen oven at 200C/400F for 25-30 minutes, or until the chicken is cooked through. Meanwhile cook the rice and peas separately in salted boiling water before combining together and serving with the chicken.

A dollop of fat-free Greek yoghurt served alongside the chicken breast makes a great addition to this meal.

Peanut Butter Chicken
Serves 1

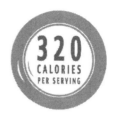

320 CALORIES PER SERVING

Ingredients:

125g/4oz skinless chicken breast
1 red (bell) pepper, sliced
½ onion, chopped
1 tbsp low fat smooth peanut butter
1 tbsp lime juice

60ml/¼ cup chicken stock
1 tsp soy sauce
1 tsp each ground cumin & coriander/cilantro
½ tsp paprika
50g/2oz boiled long grain rice
Salt & pepper to taste

Method:

Mix the ground spices and peanut butter together to form a paste. Score the chicken breast with a knife and smother in the spice paste. Add all the ingredients to an ovenproof dish and cover. Place on the lower rack and leave to cook in the halogen oven at 200C/400F for 25-30 minutes or until the chicken is cooked through. Meanwhile boil the rice in salted water until tender. Slice the chicken breast into thick slices, place on top of the rice and pour the peppers and stock over the top of the chicken.

Peanut butter is a surprisingly versatile cooking ingredient which is packed with vitamins and 'good' oils.

Parmesan Chicken & Pesto Pasta

Serves 1

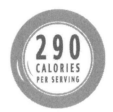

290 CALORIES PER SERVING

Ingredients:

50g/2oz fusilli pasta
1 tsp green pesto
125g/4oz skinless chicken breast

1 tsp low fat mayonnaise
2 tsp parmesan cheese, grated

Method:

Boil the pasta in salted water until tender. Drain, mix with the pesto and leave to cool. Meanwhile combine the mayonnaise & parmesan together and smother over the chicken breast. Place in an ovenproof dish on the lower rack and cook in the halogen oven at 200C/400F for 25-30 minutes or until the chicken is cooked through. Serve with the cooled pesto pasta on the side.

This is a really quick supper with which you can use any pasta or substitute for a large green and tomato salad.

Maple Chicken Wrap
Serves 1

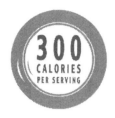

Ingredients:

125g/4oz skinless chicken breast, cubed
1 garlic clove, crushed
1 tbsp soy sauce
1 tsp maple syrup
1 tsp tomato puree/paste

½ tsp each mustard powder & ground ginger
60ml/¼ cup chicken stock
50g/2oz rocket leaves
1 tortilla wrap
Salt & pepper to taste

Method:

Mix together the stock, garlic, soy sauce, maple syrup, tomato puree and ground spices. Place the chicken pieces in an ovenproof dish and combine well with the maple syrup and stock mixture. Season well, cover and place on the lower rack of the halogen oven. Leave to cook for 25-30 minutes at 200C/400F or until the chicken is cooked through. Serve with chicken pieces in a tortilla wrap with the rocket leaves.

This is a sweet wrap which is great for a quick lunch. Use a little fat-free yoghurt if you want more creaminess to your wrap.

Chicken & Sweet Lentils
Serves 1

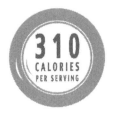

310 CALORIES PER SERVING

Ingredients:

Low-cal cooking oil spray
100g/3½oz skinless chicken
breast, sliced into strips
1 tsp each cumin & coriander
seeds, bashed with a pestle and
mortar
1 garlic clove, crushed
2 shallots, sliced

50g/2oz red lentils
1 tsp brown sugar
200g/7oz tinned chopped
tomatoes
1 tbsp tomato puree/paste
60ml/¼ cup chicken stock
50g/2oz long grain rice
Salt & pepper to taste

Method:

Gently sauté the chicken with the onion, garlic, cumin & coriander
seeds in a little low-cal oil for a few minutes. Combine all the
ingredients in an ovenproof dish, except the rice. Season well,
cover and place on the lower rack of the halogen oven. Leave
to cook for 30-35 minutes at 200C/400F or until the chicken
is cooked and the lentils are tender. Add a little more stock if
needed. Meanwhile cook the rice in salted boiling water until
tender. Serve the chicken and lentils on a bed of rice.

*Adding brown sugar to this dish gives a gentle
sweetness. Feel free to adjust this to your own taste.*

Skinny HALOGEN OVEN
BEEF, PORK & LAMB DISHES

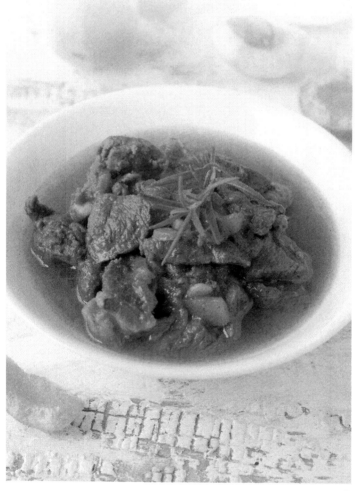

Spicy Ciabatta Quarter Pounder Burger

Serves 1

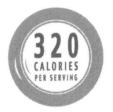

Ingredients:

Low-cal cooking oil spray
125g/4oz lean beef mince
½ piece brown bread
1 egg yolk
½ onion
1 garlic clove
1 ripe tomato, sliced

½ tsp each ground cumin, turmeric and paprika
1 tsp Dijon mustard
1 handful shredded lettuce
1 small ciabatta roll
Salt & pepper to taste

Method:

Place the bread and garlic in a food processor and pulse to make bread crumbs. Add the onion and whizz again. Add the mince, spices and egg yolk and pulse for a few seconds longer until combined. Season well and form into a large burger patty. Spray with a little low-cal cooking oil and place on the grill pan at the top of the halogen oven on 240C/475F. Grill for 5-7 mins each side, or until the burger is cooked through. Meanwhile gently toast the ciabatta roll and spread on the mustard. Serve with tomato and lettuce on top.

You could use cayenne pepper rather than paprika if you want this burger to have a 'kick'. It's worth buying a plastic burger maker to make perfect burgers shapes. They cost very little and really improve the shape and texture of the patty.

Moroccan Lamb Casserole
Serves 1

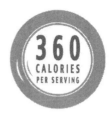

360 CALORIES PER SERVING

Ingredients:

Low-cal cooking oil spray
100g/3½oz lean lamb fillet, cubed
½ onion, chopped
1 tsp each ground cumin & coriander/cilantro
½ tsp each ground cinnamon & chilli powder
50g/2oz dried apricots, chopped

200g/7oz tinned chopped tomatoes
100g/3½oz tinned chickpeas, drained
1 garlic clove, crushed
1 tbsp worcestershire sauce
1 tbsp tomato puree/paste
1 tbsp freshly chopped flat leaf parsley
Salt & pepper to taste

Method:

Gently sauté the onion, garlic & spices in a little low-cal spray for a few minutes until softened. Add the chopped tomatoes and cubed lamb and cook for 3-4 minutes longer. Combine all the ingredients, except the chopped parsley, in an ovenproof dish. Place on the lower rack, cover and leave to cook in the halogen oven at 200C/400F for 40-50 minutes or until the lamb is tender and cooked through. Season well and serve with the chopped parsley sprinkled over the top.

The chickpeas, apricots and most importantly the spices in this Moroccan inspired dish will fill your kitchen with delicious warming smells.

37

Creamy Greek Moussaka
Serves 1

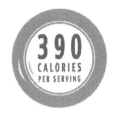

390 CALORIES PER SERVING

Ingredients:

Low-cal cooking oil spray
100g/3½oz lean lamb mince
1 small aubergine/eggplant,
halved and sliced
½ onion, chopped
½ tsp each ground cinnamon,
all spice, oregano & thyme
200g/7oz tinned chopped
tomatoes

1 garlic clove, crushed
120ml/½ cup fat free Greek
yoghurt
50g/2oz low fat grated cheddar
cheese
1 tbsp tomato puree/paste
1 tbsp freshly chopped mint
Salt & pepper to taste

Method:

Gently sauté the onion, garlic, aubergine & spices in a little low-cal oil for a few minutes until the aubergine is nicely softened. Add the chopped tomatoes, puree and lamb mince and cook for 3-4 minutes longer. Place all the ingredients, except the chopped mint, yoghurt and cheese, in an ovenproof dish. Meanwhile very gently heat the yoghurt and cheese together in a saucepan and, when combined, carefully pour over the top of the casserole dish.

Place on the lower rack, cover and leave to cook in the halogen oven at 200C/400F for 25-30 minutes or until the lamb is tender and cooked through. Season well and serve with the chopped mint sprinkled over the top.

Mousakka is popular in both Balkan and Mediterranean cuisine. Using Greek yoghurt rather than a traditional 'white' sauce topping cuts down considerably on the calories of this dish.

Wiltshire Ham & Mustard Leeks
Serves 1

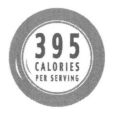

395 CALORIES PER SERVING

Ingredients:

Low-cal cooking oil spray
1 tsp low-cal 'butter' spread
1 tsp plain/all-purpose flour
120ml/½ cup semi skimmed milk
100g/3½oz potatoes, peeled & cubed
25g/1oz grated low fat cheese
½ tsp each dijon & wholegrain mustard

1 leek, sliced
100g/3 ½oz lean Wiltshire-cured ham, chopped
2 tbsp breadcrumbs
1 clove garlic
1 tbsp freshly chopped parsley
75g/3oz tenderstem broccoli, roughly chopped
Salt & pepper to taste

Method:

Gently sauté the garlic, potatoes & leek in a little low-cal spray for a few minutes until softened. Gently heat the 'butter' in a saucepan and add the flour, stirring continuously to create a roux. Slowly add the milk and carry on stirring to prevent lumps. Warm through until the sauce thickens a little. Combine all the ingredients in an ovenproof dish and sprinkle the breadcrumbs on top. Place on the lower rack and leave to cook in the halogen oven at 200C/400F for 15-20 minutes or until the vegetables are tender. Season well and serve.

A roux is just a creamy paste which is made using butter and flour - the trick is to keep on stirring.

Italian Basil Meatballs & Spaghetti
Serves 1

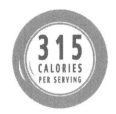

Ingredients:

Low-cal cooking oil spray
100g/3½ oz lean beef mince
½ piece brown bread
1 egg yolk
½ onion
1 garlic clove
½ tsp each ground cumin,
turmeric and paprika

1 tsp dried oregano
2 tbsp freshly chopped basil
250ml/1 cup tomato passatta/
sieved tomatoes
1 tbsp worcestershire sauce
½ tsp each salt & brown sugar
50g/2oz spaghetti
Salt & pepper to taste

Method:

Place the bread and garlic in a food processor and pulse to make bread crumbs. Add the onion and whizz again. Add the mince, spices, herbs and egg yolk and pulse for a few seconds longer until well combined. Season and form into small meatballs with your hands.

Place on an oven proof dish, spray with a little low cal-cooking oil and put on the lower rack in the halogen oven at 200C/400F for 10-15 minutes. Meanwhile combine together the passatta, worcestershire sauce, salt & sugar. Add to the meatballs, mix well and continue to cook for a further 10-15 minutes until the meatballs are cooked through and the sauce is piping hot. Meanwhile cook the spaghetti in salted boiling water until tender. Serve with the meatballs and sauce piled on top of the spaghetti.

Meatballs are a staple of Italian food which have become a firm family favourite in the UK & US. Serve with grated parmesan cheese and a salad if you like.

Creamy Sirloin Stroganoff & Pappardelle
Serves 1

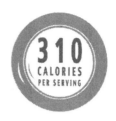

310 CALORIES PER SERVING

Ingredients:

Low-cal cooking oil spray
125g/4oz lean sirloin steak, cut into fine strips
½ onion, chopped
½ tsp each oregano & tarragon
75g/3oz chestnut mushrooms, sliced

1 garlic clove, crushed
1 tsp dijon mustard
60ml/¼ cup beef stock
2 tbsp low fat crème fraiche
50g/2oz pappardelle pasta
Salt & pepper to taste

Method:

Gently sauté the onion, garlic & mushrooms in a little low-cal oil for a few minutes. Add the steak and cook for 3-4 minutes longer. Place all the ingredients, except the pasta, in an ovenproof dish and combine well. Place on the lower rack, cover and leave to cook in the halogen oven at 200C/400F for 10-15 minutes or until the sauce is creamy & the steak is tender and cooked through (add a little more crème fraiche if needed). Meanwhile cook the pappardelle in salted boiling water until tender. Season well and serve with the stroganoff piled on top of the pasta.

Rice is traditionally served with stroganoff but this version used thick pappardelle ribbons which make a really hearty meal. Try putting the steak in the freezer for half an hour before slicing and you'll find it easier to cut it into very fine strips which will be more tender in the meal.

Sausage & Chorizo Casserole
Serves 1

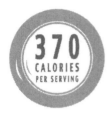

370 CALORIES PER SERVING

Ingredients:

Low-cal cooking oil spray
50g/2oz lean pork sausages, sliced
50g/2oz uncooked chorizo sausages, sliced
½ onion, chopped
1 red (bell) pepper, sliced
1 tsp each mixed dried herbs & smoked paprika

200g/7oz tinned chopped tomatoes
100g/3½oz tinned mixed beans, drained
2 garlic cloves, crushed
1 tbsp worcestershire sauce
1 tbsp tomato puree/paste
Salt & pepper to taste

Method:

Gently sauté the onion, sliced pepper, garlic & herbs in a little low-cal oil for a few minutes until softened. Add the sausages and chorizo and cook for 3-4 minutes longer. Combine all the ingredients in an ovenproof dish. Place on the lower rack and leave to cook in the halogen oven at 200C/400F for 25-30 minutes or until the sausages are cooked through and the beans are tender. Season well and serve.

Chorizo sausage comes as either a cooked 'salami' type sausage or as an uncooked sausage which must be cooked before eating. Use the uncooked variety for this dish.

Apple Cider Pork With Garlic Mushrooms

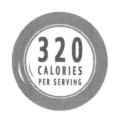

320 CALORIES PER SERVING

Serves 1

Ingredients:

Low-cal cooking oil spray
125g/4oz pork loin steak
60ml/¼ cup dry cider
1 eating apple, peeled & chopped
2 garlic cloves, crushed

75g/3oz mushrooms, sliced
1 tbsp crème fraiche
75g/3oz shredded vegetable ribbons
Salt & pepper to taste

Method:

Season the pork loin. Spray with a little low-cal cooking oil and place in an ovenproof dish on the grill pan at the top of the halogen oven at 240C/475F. Grill for 3-4 mins each side. Meanwhile gently sauté the chopped apple, garlic and mushrooms in a little low-cal oil for a few minutes until softened. Stir through the cider and crème fraiche and pour over the pork steak (use the same pan for the vegetables later). Reduce the heat in the halogen oven to 200C/400F and cook for a further 4-6 minutes or until the pork is cooked through. Meanwhile use the same pan to gently sauté the vegetable ribbons for a few minutes in any leftover juices from the mushroom mixture.

Pan-ready prepared shredded vegetables are widely available and really useful to have in. Or use a beansprout/vegetable stir-fry pack.

Citrus & Sage Pork Fillet
Serves 1

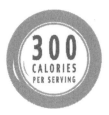

300 CALORIES PER SERVING

Ingredients:

Low-cal cooking oil spray
125g/4oz piece pork tenderloin
60ml/¼ cup chicken stock
1 orange, juiced
1 garlic clove, crushed
1 tbsp freshly chopped sage

75g/3oz butternut squash, peeled & cut into thin chips or small cubes
50g/2oz spinach, chopped
Salt & pepper to taste

Method:

Season the pork tenderloin. Spray with a little low-cal cooking oil and quickly brown all over in a frying pan for a few minutes. Place in an ovenproof dish with all the other ingredients and cover tightly. Cook on the lower rack of the halogen oven at 200C/400F for 25-30 minutes or until the pork is cooked through and the squash is tender. Remove the pork and cut into thick slices. Arrange on the plate with the spinach and squash to the side. Pour the stock and orange juices over the top of the pork and vegetables and serve.

Root vegetables can take longer to cook than meat so ensure the squash is cut into small enough pieces so that it is tender once the pork is cooked.

Chocolate Chilli
Serves 1

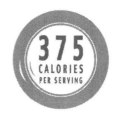

Ingredients:

Low-cal cooking oil spray
125g/4oz lean minced beef
1 tsp each ground cumin & mild chilli powder
2 tsp cocoa powder
½ tsp ground allspice
1 carrot, cut into batons
½ onion, chopped

1 garlic clove, crushed
1 tsp each dried basil
2 tsp sundried tomato paste
60ml/¼ cup beef stock
2 taco shells
1 tbsp fat-free Greek yoghurt
1 handful shredded lettuce
Salt & pepper to taste

Method:

Gently sauté the onion, garlic, spices & herbs in a little low-cal spray for a few minutes until softened. Add all the other ingredients and cook for 2-3 minutes longer. Combine all the ingredients in an ovenproof dish. Place on the lower rack and leave to cook in the halogen oven at 200C/400F for 15-20 minutes or until the mince is cooked through. Season well and serve with the taco shells, shredded lettuce and yoghurt.

Load the chocolate mince into each taco shell and arrange the lettuce and yoghurt on top. Messy but delicious!

Indian Minted Lamb & Carrots
Serves 1

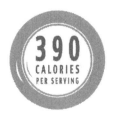

Ingredients:

Low-cal cooking oil spray
125g/4oz lean lamb fillet, cubed
2 tbsp balsamic vinegar
½ tsp each garam masala, ground turmeric, coriander/cilantro
1 garlic clove, crushed

2 carrots, chopped
½ red onion, chopped
1 tsp mint sauce
60ml/¼ cup lamb or chicken stock
1 chapatti bread
Salt & pepper to taste

Method:

Season the lamb, spray with a little low-cal cooking oil and quickly brown all over in a frying pan for a few minutes. Place in an ovenproof dish with all the other ingredients and cover tightly. Cook on the lower rack of the halogen oven at 200C/400F for 30-35 minutes or until the lamb is cooked through and the carrots are tender. Serve with the chapatti bread on the side.

Chapatti is a light Indian bread ideal for mopping up the delicious cooking juices. It is readily available in most supermarkets but you could also use pitta bread.

Shami Tikka
Serves 1

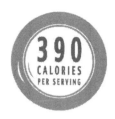

390 CALORIES PER SERVING

Ingredients:

Low-cal cooking oil spray
125g/4oz lean lamb mince
½ tsp each ground coriander,
garlic, salt, paprika, cumin &
turmeric
½ onion, very finely chopped
1 green chilli, very finely
chopped

1 tbsp freshly chopped mint
1 tsp lemon juice
1 small pitta bread
1 handful shredded lettuce
1 vine ripened tomato, finely
chopped
Salt & pepper to taste

Method:

Gently sauté the onion, green chillies, coriander, paprika, cumin,
turmeric and garlic in a little low-cal cooking oil for a few minutes.
Place the mince, lemon juice, chopped mint and warm spicy
onion mixture into a food processor and whizz together. Take
the mixture out, divide into 5-6 portions and shape into small
flat meat patties. Spray with a little low-cal cooking oil and place
on the grill pan at the top of the halogen oven on 240C/475F.
Grill for 4-5 minutes each side or until the lamb is properly
cooked through. Serve inside the pitta bread with the lettuce and
tomatoes.

*Shami Tikka is a traditional Indian starter which
differs from Sheik Kebab with its flat patties and
inclusion of paprika, turmeric and cumin.*

Sweet Sesame Seed Pork & Noodles
Serves 1

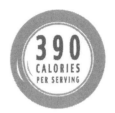

390 CALORIES PER SERVING

Ingredients:

Low-cal cooking oil spray
125g/4oz pork tenderloin, cubed
½ onion, chopped
1 garlic clove, crushed
1 tsp runny honey
2 tsp tomato puree/paste
60ml/¼ cup chicken stock

1 tsp sesame seeds
1 small bunch chopped spring onions/scallions
½ pak choi, shredded
½ lime, cut into wedges
50g/2oz cooked egg noodles
Salt & pepper to taste

Method:

Season the pork, spray with a little low-cal cooking oil and quickly brown all over in a frying pan for a few minutes. Place in an ovenproof dish with all the other ingredients, except the sesame seeds, spring onions, lime wedges and noodles. Cover tightly and cook on the lower rack of the halogen oven at 200C/400F for 20-25 minutes or until the pork is cooked through. Serve on a bed of cooked noodles with the sesame seeds and spring onions sprinkled over the top and lime wedges on the side.

The honey gives a sweetness to this dish which is lifted at the end with spring onions and lime juices as a garnish. Pour any leftover juices over the top of the pork and noodles.

Sausage & Spinach Gnocchi
Serves 1

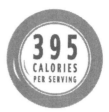

395 CALORIES PER SERVING

Ingredients:

Low-cal cooking oil spray
2 lean pork sausages, sliced
½ onion, chopped
1 tbsp worcestershire sauce
60ml/¼ cup passata/sieved tomatoes

1 tsp dried rosemary
Pinch salt & brown sugar
100g/3½oz tinned chopped tomatoes
50g/2oz fresh spinach
125g/4oz gnocchi

Method:

Gently brown the onion and sliced sausages in a little low-cal cooking oil for a few minutes. Place in an ovenproof dish with all the ingredients and mix well. Cover and cook on the lower rack of the halogen oven at 200C/400F for 15-20 minutes or until the sausages are cooked through and the gnocchi dumplings are tender.

Use the salt & sugar to balance the acidity of the tomatoes in this dish, a small pinch of both should be enough.

Liver & Onions
Serves 1

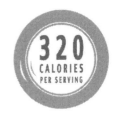

320 CALORIES PER SERVING

Ingredients:

Low-cal cooking oil spray
125g/4oz liver, sliced
2 onions, sliced
60ml/¼ cup chicken stock
1 tbsp low fat crème fraiche

½ tsp paprika
1 tbsp freshly chopped flat leaf parsley
1 slice thick granary bread, lightly toasted

Method:

Gently brown the onions and liver slices in a little low-cal cooking oil for a few minutes. Place in an ovenproof dish with the stock, parsley & crème fraiche. Mix well, cover and cook on the lower rack of the halogen oven at 180C/350F for 30-40 minutes or until the liver is cooked through and the onions are tender. Pile on top of the granary bread, sprinkle with paprika and serve.

You could also add some sliced mushrooms and a side salad to this meal if you wanted to bulk it out a little.

Skinny HALOGEN OVEN

FISH & SEAFOOD DISHES

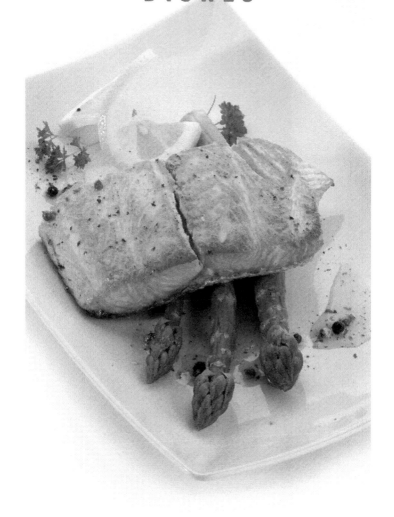

Lemon Sole & Garlic Breadcrumbs
Serves 1

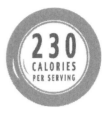

230 CALORIES PER SERVING

Ingredients:

Low-cal cooking oil spray
125g/4oz skinless, boneless lemon sole fillet
1 garlic clove, crushed
½ onion, chopped
2 tbsp fresh breadcrumbs
1 tbsp freshly chopped flat leaf parsley

50g/2oz chestnut mushrooms, chopped
2 vine ripened tomatoes
1 tsp anchovy paste
50g/2oz rocket leaves
½ lemon cut into wedges
Salt & pepper to taste

Method:

Slice the lemon sole fillet to create a cavity for stuffing. Gently sauté the mushrooms, garlic, onions & anchovy paste together in a little low-cal oil for a few minutes. Stuff this mixture into the fillet. Mix together the breadcrumbs and chopped parsley. Place the stuffed fillet and tomatoes on the grill pan of the halogen oven, season and sprinkle with the breadcrumb mix. Cook for 8-12 minutes at 240C/475F or until the fish is properly cooked through. Serve with the rocket salad and lemon wedges.

Although strong in taste, the anchovy paste and peppery rocket salad in this dish are careful not to overpower the delicate flavour of the lemon sole.

Pesto Salmon & Crushed Sweet Potatoes

Serves 1

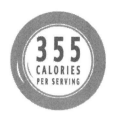

355 CALORIES PER SERVING

Ingredients:

125g/4oz thick skinless, boneless salmon fillet
2 tsp green pesto
1 tbsp fresh breadcrumbs

125g/4oz sweet potato, peeled & cubed
50g/2oz mangetout
Salt & pepper to taste

Method:

Mix together the breadcrumbs and pesto and spread over the top of the salmon fillet. Place the salmon on the grill pan at the top of the halogen oven and cook for 8-12 minutes at 240C/475F or until the salmon is properly cooked through. Meanwhile boil the sweet potato for 10 minutes or until tender. Season well and mash a little with the back of a fork. Steam the mangetout for a few minutes on top of the boiling pan while the potatoes are cooking. Arrange the vegetables and fish together on a plate and serve.

Shop-bought pesto in a jar is perfect for this recipe and complements the naturally oily nature of the salmon.

53

Sweet Sesame Salmon & Asparagus

Serves 1

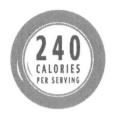

240 CALORIES PER SERVING

Ingredients:

125g/4oz thick skinless, boneless salmon fillet
1 tsp runny honey
1 tsp soy sauce

½ tsp sesame oil
½ lemon cut into wedges
75g/3oz asparagus spears
Salt & pepper to taste

Method:

Mix together the honey, soy sauce and sesame oil. Place the salmon and asparagus on the grill pan at the top of the halogen oven and brush with the honey mix. Cook for 8-12 minutes at 240C/475F or until the salmon is properly cooked through and the asparagus are tender. Serve with lemon wedges on the side.

Use a thick piece of salmon for this recipe. You could add a pinch of crushed chillies to the asparagus spears for an extra 'bite' too.

Balsamic Tuna Steak
Serves 1

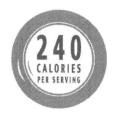

240 CALORIES PER SERVING

Ingredients:

125g/4oz thick boneless tuna fillet
1 tsp balsamic vinegar
1 tsp soy sauce

½ tsp chilli oil
125g/4oz beansprout & vegetable mix
Salt & pepper to taste

Method:

Mix together the balsamic vinegar, soy sauce and chilli oil. Place the tuna on the grill pan at the top of the halogen oven and brush with the balsamic/oil mix. Cook for 6-10 minutes at 240C/475F or until the tuna is cooked to your preference (6 minutes of cooking will leave it quite rare). Meanwhile use the rest of the balsamic/oil mix to stir-fry the beansprouts for a few minutes while the tuna cooks in the halogen oven. Add a little more soy sauce to the beansprouts during cooking if needed. Serve the tuna steak on top of the stir-fried beansprouts and vegetables.

Bags of fresh beansprouts and shredded vegetables are available almost everywhere and are really quick and easy to use.

Tuna & Noodle Bake
Serves 1

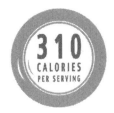

310 CALORIES PER SERVING

Ingredients:

Low-cal cooking oil spray
1 onion, chopped
125g/4oz tinned tuna, drained
50g/2oz sugar snap peas,
roughly chopped
75g/3oz cooked fine egg
noodles

200g/7oz tinned chopped
tomatoes
½ tsp crushed chilli flakes
1 tbsp sundried tomato paste
Salt & pepper to taste

Method:

Gently sauté the onion in a little low-cal spray for a few minutes until soft. Combine all the ingredients really well in an ovenproof dish. Place on the lower rack and leave to cook in the halogen oven at 200C/400F for 20-25 minutes or until piping hot.

This dish will work just as well with pasta rather than noodles. Increase the chilli to your own taste and add grated parmesan cheese if you like.

Tandoori & Pepper, Prawn Kebabs
Serves 1

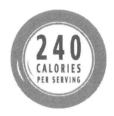

240 CALORIES PER SERVING

Ingredients:

Low-cal cooking oil spray
125g/4oz large raw king prawns
1 tsp each ground cumin,
turmeric, coriander/cilantro &
chilli powder
½ tsp each ground ginger &
garam masala
1 tbsp lemon juice
2 garlic cloves, crushed

1 baby gem lettuce, shredded
1 large (bell) pepper, cut into
pieces
½ lemon cut into wedges
2 tbsp fat-free Greek yoghurt
1 tsp mint sauce
3 metal skewers
Salt & pepper to taste

Method:

Mix together the lemon juice, ground spices & garlic to form a paste (add a little water if needed). Season the prawns and pepper pieces, spray with a little low-cal oil and smother in the spice paste. Place in an ovenproof dish and leave for up to 1 hour to marinate.

Skewer the prawns and pepper pieces in turn to make two or three kebabs. Place on the grill pan at the top of the halogen oven on 240C/475F. Grill for 4-6 minutes each side or until the prawns are cooked through and the pepper pieces are tender (take care handling the skewers as they will get hot).

Meanwhile mix the mint sauce and Greek yoghurt together. Plate up the skewers along with the shredded lettuce and serve the lemon wedges and mint yoghurt on the side.

Any type of large raw prawn is good for this dish, use peeled or unpeeled depending on your own preference.

Creamy Cod & Broccoli Bake
Serves 1

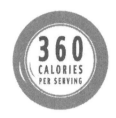

360 CALORIES PER SERVING

Ingredients:

2 tbsp fresh breadcrumbs
75g/3oz small peeled prawns
75g/3oz boneless cod fillet, cut into chunks
50g/2oz spinach, chopped
50g/2oz tenderstem broccoli, roughly chopped

50g/2oz sweetcorn
60ml/¼ cup milk
1 tbsp low fat soft cream cheese
½ lemon cut into wedges
Salt & pepper to taste

Method:

Gently heat the milk and cream cheese in a saucepan to make a creamy sauce. Combine all the ingredients in an ovenproof dish, season and sprinkle the breadcrumbs on top. Place on the lower rack and leave to cook in the halogen oven at 200C/400F for 20-25 minutes or until the seafood is properly cooked through and the vegetables are tender. Serve with lemon wedges on the side.

To make fresh breadcrumbs put a slice of bread and a little seasoning in a food processor and pulse for a few seconds.

Mediterranean Fish Stew
Serves 1

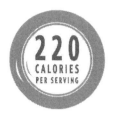

220 CALORIES PER SERVING

Ingredients:

75g/3oz small peeled prawns
75g/3oz boneless meaty white fish, cut into chunks
1 onion, chopped
1 garlic clove, crushed
60ml/¼ cup fish or chicken stock
125g/4oz fresh tomatoes, finely chopped

1 tsp anchovy paste
Splash dry white wine
1 tbsp sundried tomato paste
1 tbsp each freshly chopped rosemary & basil
1 bay leaf
Salt & pepper to taste

Method:

Gently sauté the onion, anchovy paste & garlic in a little low-cal oil for a few minutes. Add all the ingredients to an ovenproof dish and season well. Cover with foil, place on the lower rack and leave to cook in the halogen oven at 180C/350F for 30-35 minutes or until the seafood is properly cooked through.

This fish dish is lovely served with freshly baked crusty bread to soak up all the tasty juices.

Pollack & Tahini Sauce
Serves 1

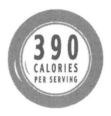

390 CALORIES PER SERVING

Ingredients:

125g/4oz skinless, boneless pollack fillet
1 tsp tahini paste
1 tbsp soy sauce
2 tbsp freshly chopped coriander/cilantro

2 large vine ripened tomatoes, sliced
½ red onion sliced into rounds
125g/4oz tinned kidney beans, drained
Salt & pepper to taste

Method:

Mix together the tahini paste, soy sauce and 1 tbsp of the chopped coriander. Place the pollack fillet on the grill pan at the top of the halogen oven and brush over the tahini & herb mixture. Cook for 8-12 minutes at 240C/475F or until the fish is properly cooked through.

Meanwhile arrange the kidney beans, sliced tomatoes and onion slices on a plate. Scatter the remaining chopped coriander over the top. Season and serve with the cooked pollack fillet.

Pollack is a superb meaty fish but any firm white fish fillet will do well with this recipe. Add fresh parsley too if you have it.

Whole Stuffed Sardines & Potato Salad

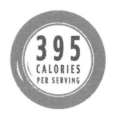

395 CALORIES PER SERVING

Serves 1

Ingredients:

Low-cal cooking oil spray
200g/7oz whole fresh sardines, gutted and cleaned
1 garlic clove, crushed
½ onion, chopped
2 tbsp fresh breadcrumbs
1 tbsp freshly chopped flat leaf parsley
1 tsp capers, chopped

1 tsp sultanas, chopped
125g/4oz salad potatoes, halved
1 small bunch spring onions/ scallions, chopped.
1 tsp low-fat mayonnaise
½ lemon cut into wedges
Salt & pepper to taste

Method:

First make a simple potato salad by boiling the salad potatoes in salted water until tender. Season well, leave to cool and mix with the mayonnaise & spring onions.

Gently sauté the garlic, breadcrumbs, capers and sultanas in a little low-cal oil for a few minutes until softened. Stuff the breadcrumb/caper mix into the whole sardines and place on the grill pan of the halogen oven. Season and cook for 8-12 minutes at 240C/475F or until the fish is properly cooked through. Sprinkle chopped parsley over the top and serve with the potato salad and lemon wedges at the side.

Any fishmonger will be happy to gut and clean fresh sardines to make ready for stuffing and cooking.

Store Cupboard Sardines
Serves 1

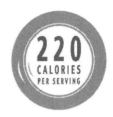

220 CALORIES PER SERVING

Ingredients:

1 slice wholegrain brown bread
100g/3½oz tinned boneless
sardines in tomato sauce

½ tsp paprika
2 tsp chopped capers or olives
Salt & pepper to taste

Method:

Gently toast the bread. Mash the sardines a little with the back of a fork to break up the fillets and add the capers or olives. Spread over the toast and sprinkle with paprika. Place on the grill pan of the halogen oven and cook for 3-4 minutes at 240C/475F or piping hot.

If you are looking for a super-simple supper this is an easy option and tinned sardines are a fantastic source of omega-3 fatty acids, calcium, iron and potassium.

Lime Monkfish & Crushed Potatoes
Serves 1

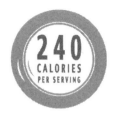

Ingredients:

Low-cal cooking oil spray
125g/4oz monkfish fillets
75g/3oz salad potatoes
1 orange (bell) pepper, sliced
½ red onion, sliced

1 tsp freshly chopped
coriander/cilantro
3 tbsp lime juice
50g/2 oz salad leaves
Salt & pepper to taste

Method:

Gently cook the potatoes in salted boiling water until tender. Season, crush gently with a fork and sprinkle with the chopped coriander. Meanwhile combine the monkfish, peppers and onions with the lime juice and leave to marinate for a few minutes. Season, place on a grill tray at the top of the halogen oven and cook for 8-12 minutes at 240C/475F or until the fish is properly cooked through and the vegetables are tender. Serve the monkfish, and vegetables with the crushed potatoes and salad leaves on the side.

The lime juice not only marinates the monkfish it also begins to 'cook' the fillet so don't leave it to marinate for too long.

Skinny HALOGEN OVEN

VEGETABLE/VEGETARIAN DISHES

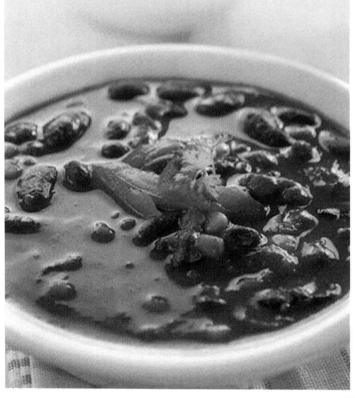

Roasted Pepper & Garlic Warm Salad

Serves 1

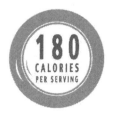

Ingredients:

Low-cal cooking oil spray
1 red (bell) pepper, sliced
1 tbsp balsamic vinegar
100g/3½oz vine ripened
tomatoes, halved

2 garlic cloves, crushed
½ red onion, chopped
1 tbsp freshly chopped basil
100g/3½oz mixed leaf salad
Salt & pepper to taste

Method:

Mix together the balsamic vinegar with the onions, garlic, peppers and tomatoes. Place in an ovenproof dish and spray with a little low-cal oil. Place on the lower rack and leave to cook in the halogen oven at 180C/350F for 30-40 minutes or until the vegetables are tender. Season well and serve tossed through the salad leaves with the chopped basil sprinkled over the top. Pour any juices on the salad as a dressing.

You could add a pinch of brown sugar to the tomatoes to slightly caramelise during cooking in the halogen.

Wholemeal Pitta Pizza

Serves 1

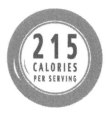

Ingredients:

Low-cal cooking oil spray
1 wholemeal pitta bread
2 tsp sundried tomato paste
1 vine ripened tomato, chopped
½ red onion, chopped
25g/1oz low fat cheddar cheese, grated

1 tbsp freshly chopped basil leaves
Handful spinach leaves, chopped
1 baby gem lettuce, shredded
Salt & pepper to taste

Method:

Slice the pitta bread lengthways to make two halves. Use only one half for this recipe as a pizza base. Spread the sundried paste over the base. Arrange the tomatoes, onion, cheese, basil and spinach leaves on the pitta. Spray with a little low-cal cooking oil and place on the grill pan of the halogen oven on the top shelf at 220C/425F. Grill for 8-10 minutes or until the pizza is cooked through. Serve with shredded lettuce on the side.

There are any number of toppings you could use on your pitta pizza, feel free to experiment with your own favourites.

Baked Garlic & Tomato Portabella Mushroom

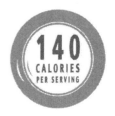

Serves 1

Ingredients:

Low-cal cooking oil spray
1 large portabella mushroom
1 vine ripened tomato, chopped
25g/1oz low fat mozzarella cheese, chopped

1 tbsp chopped chives
75g/3oz asparagus spears
Salt & pepper to taste

Method:

Mix together the chopped tomato, cheese & chives. Spray the mushroom and asparagus with a little low cal-cooking oil, season well and place on the grill pan at the top of the halogen oven. Pile the tomato mix on top of the mushroom and grill at 220C/425F for 10-12 minutes or until the mushroom and asparagus are tender and cooked through.

Mushrooms and asparagus are a lovely combination. Add a little more cooking spray if needed during cooking and cover the mushroom to prevent burning.

Red Cabbage Casserole

Serves 1

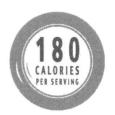

180 CALORIES PER SERVING

Ingredients:

Low-cal cooking oil spray
1 onion, chopped
250g/9oz red cabbage, shredded
1 tsp fennel seeds
1 tbsp horseradish sauce

1 tsp caraway seeds
1 eating apple, peeled & chopped
120ml/½ cup fat free Greek yoghurt
Salt & pepper to taste

Method:

Gently sauté the onion, fennel & caraway seeds in a little low-cal spray for a few minutes until softened. Combine all the ingredients in an ovenproof dish, place on the lower rack, cover and leave to cook in the halogen oven at 200C/400F for 40-50 minutes or until the vegetables are tender and cooked through.

You could use fresh fennel rather than fennel seeds if you prefer, you may also like to add a little chopped lean bacon if you are not vegetarian.

Mozzarella Baked Baby Vegetables
Serves 1

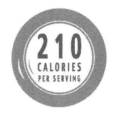

Ingredients:

Low-cal cooking oil spray
1 red (bell) pepper, sliced
2 garlic cloves, crushed
50g/2oz cherry tomatoes
50g/2oz baby sweetcorn
50g/2oz shallots
50g/2oz aubergines or courgettes/zucchini

50g/2oz pitted olives, chopped
2 tbsp freshly chopped basil
25g/1oz low fat mozzarella cheese, chopped
Salt & pepper to taste

Method:

Combine all the ingredients, except the chopped basil, in an ovenproof dish. Place on the lower rack, cover and leave to cook in the halogen oven at 180C/350F for 40-50 minutes or until the vegetables are tender and cooked through.

Any mix of baby vegetables will work fine for this recipe. Serve as a main course for one or side dish for two.

Green Lentil & Bean Bake

Serves

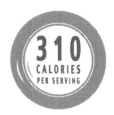

310 CALORIES PER SERVING

Ingredients:

Low-cal cooking oil spray
1 leek, thinly sliced
1 garlic clove, crushed
50g/2oz courgettes/zucchini
50g/2oz green beans, chopped
25g/1oz sundried tomatoes, chopped

25g/1oz pitted olives, chopped
40g/1½oz green lentils
120ml/½ cup vegetable stock
1 tbsp freshly chopped flat leaf parsley
Salt & pepper to taste

Method:

Gently sauté the leek and garlic in a little low-cal oil for a few minutes until softened. Combine all the ingredients, except the chopped parsley, in an ovenproof dish. Place on the lower rack, cover and leave to cook in the halogen oven at 180C/350F for 40-50 minutes or until the lentils are tender and cooked through. Add a little more stock if needed during cooking to ensure the lentils are tender.

Just before serving add a squeeze of lemon juice if you have it.

Tarka-Dhal
Serves 1

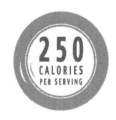

Ingredients:

Low-cal cooking oil spray
25g/1oz yellow split peas
25g/1oz red lentils
1 carrot, chopped
120ml/½ cup vegetable stock
1 garlic cloves, crushed
1 fresh tomatoes, chopped
1 tsp ground turmeric
1 red chilli, deseeded and finely chopped

1 onion, chopped
½ tsp each mustard seeds & onions seeds
½ tsp crushed chilli flakes
1 tbsp freshly chopped coriander/cilantro
1 tbsp lime juice
Salt & pepper to taste

Method:

Gently sauté the onions and garlic in a little low-cal spray for a few minutes until softened. Combine all the ingredients, except the chopped coriander and lime juice, in an ovenproof dish. Place on the lower rack, cover and leave to cook in the halogen oven at 180C/350F for 40-50 minutes or until the lentils and peas are cooked through. Add a little more stock if needed during cooking to ensure the lentils are tender. Stir through the lime juice and sprinkle over the chopped coriander before serving.

A dollop of fat free Greek yoghurt is great with this dish. You could stir a little mint sauce through it to make a superfast raita.

Ditalini & Borlotti Beans
Serves 1

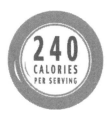

Ingredients:

Low-cal cooking oil spray
125g/4oz tinned borlotti beans
50g/2oz ditalini pasta
1 tsp dried rosemary
2 garlic cloves, crushed

1 tbsp tomato puree/paste
½ onion, chopped
60ml/¼ cup vegetable stock
Salt & pepper to taste

Method:

Cook the pasta in salted boiling water until tender. Combine all the ingredients in an ovenproof dish. Place on the lower rack, cover and leave to cook in the halogen oven at 200C/400F for 20-25 minutes or until the pasta and beans are piping hot and cooked through.

Ditalini is a short macaroni style pasta. Feel free to substitute with any other similar small soup pasta.

Pak Choi Broth
Serves 1

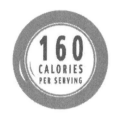

Ingredients:

250ml/1 cup vegetable stock
75g/3oz pak choi, sliced
25g/1oz purple sprouting
broccoli, roughly chopped
25g/1oz potatoes, peeled & cut
into very small cubes
25g/1oz fresh peas

2 shallots, chopped
1 tsp brown sugar
½ leek, chopped
1 tsp freshly grated ginger
½ tsp crushed chilli flakes
1 garlic clove, crushed
Salt & pepper to taste

Method:

Combine all the ingredients in an oven proof dish. Place on
the lower rack, cover and leave to cook in the halogen oven at
180C/350F for 35-40 minutes or until the vegetables are tender.

*Pak choi is a fantastic Asian vegetable which is
versatile and surprisingly easy to grow even in some
of the toughest climates. To make this more of a soup
you should double the stock quantities.*

Eastern Stew
Serves 1

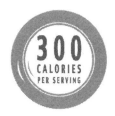

Ingredients:

60ml/¼ cup vegetable stock
1 green (bell) pepper, sliced
1 carrot, chopped
1 courgette/zucchini, sliced
2 celery stalks, chopped
50g/2oz sweet potato, peeled & cubed
200g/7oz tinned chopped tomatoes

200g/7oz tinned chickpeas
1 tsp each mild chilli powder & ground cumin
2 garlic cloves, crushed
1 tsp freshly chopped mint
Salt & pepper to taste

Method:

Combine all the ingredients, except the mint, in an ovenproof dish. Place on the lower rack, cover and leave to cook in the halogen oven at 200C/400F for 25-30 minutes or until the vegetables are tender. Season, sprinkle with chopped mint and serve.

This is a great main course which you can serve as it is, or with some tender couscous and a twist of lemon juice.

Simple Spanish Tortilla
Serves 1

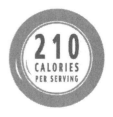

210 CALORIES PER SERVING

Ingredients:

Low-cal cooking oil spray
1 onion
100g/3½oz potatoes, leave
unpeeled

1 large free range egg
50g/2oz mixed salad leaves
Salt & pepper to taste

Method:

In a food processor whizz together the potatoes and onion. Gently
sauté in a little low-cal oil for a 5-10 minutes until softened. Beat
the egg and combine with the sautéed mixture in a small greased
ovenproof dish. Season well, place on the lower rack and cook
in the halogen oven at 200C/400F for 20-25 minutes or until the
omelette is firm. Serve with mixed salad leaves on the side.

*This is a simple Spanish dish which is often served in
thick slices as tapas. If you are not vegetarian you
could add some sliced chorizo sausage at the sauté
stage of cooking.*

Paneer & Pepper Kebabs
Serves 1

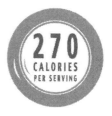

270 CALORIES PER SERVING

Ingredients:

Low-cal cooking oil spray
75g/3oz paneer cheese, cubed
50g/2oz cooked salad potatoes
1 red (bell) pepper, cut into cubes
1 red onion, cut into wedges
1 tsp each ground cumin, turmeric, coriander/cilantro & chilli powder
½ tsp each ground ginger & garam masala

1 tbsp lemon juice
2 garlic cloves, crushed
1 baby gem lettuce, shredded
½ lemon cut into wedges
2 tbsp fat free Greek yoghurt
1 tsp mint sauce
2 metal skewers
Salt & pepper to taste

Method:

Mix together the lemon juice, ground spices & garlic to form a paste and combine with the yoghurt. Add the cheese, onion, pepper and potato pieces to the yoghurt and combine. Season and leave to marinate for up to an hour.

Skewer the pieces to make two vegetable kebabs. Place on the grill pan at the top of the halogen oven at 240C/475F and cook for 6-8 minutes each side or until the vegetables are tender and the cheese is cooked through. Serve with the shredded lettuce and lemon wedges.

Paneer is a commonly used cheese in Indian cooking. It can be bought in balls or in cubes - which are easiest for this recipe.

Light Macaroni Cheese
Serves 1

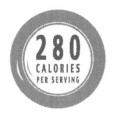

280 CALORIES PER SERVING

Ingredients:

75g/3oz macaroni pasta
1 tsp Dijon mustard
60ml/¼ cup low fat crème fraiche
2 tbsp milk
Pinch nutmeg

50g/2oz grated mature cheddar cheese
25g/1oz spinach, chopped
2 vine ripened tomatoes, chopped
Salt & pepper to taste

Method:

Cook the pasta in salted boiling water until tender. Meanwhile gently warm through the mustard, crème fraiche, milk, nutmeg and cheese in a saucepan. Combine all the ingredients in an ovenproof dish. Season well, cover and place on the lower rack of the halogen oven. Leave to cook for 25-30 minutes at 200C/400F or until piping hot.

Wholegrain mustard is also good in this recipe. You could also substitute some steamed tenderstem broccoli in place of the spinach.

Vegetable & Bean Chilli

Serves 1

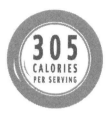

305
CALORIES
PER SERVING

Ingredients:

Low-cal cooking oil spray
1 onion, chopped
200g/7oz tinned chopped tomatoes
200g/7oz tinned mixed beans
1 tbsp tomato puree/paste
25g/1oz chestnut mushrooms, sliced
1 carrot, chopped

1 red chilli, chopped
½ tsp crushed chilli flakes
1 tsp each ground cumin, paprika & coriander/cilantro
1 garlic clove, crushed
1 tsp brown sugar
1 tbsp freshly chopped coriander/cilantro
Salt & pepper to taste

Method:

Gently sauté the onion, garlic and mushroom in a little low-cal oil until softened. Combine all the ingredients, except the chopped coriander, in an ovenproof dish. Season well, cover and place on the lower rack of the halogen oven. Leave to cook for 25-30 minutes at 200C/400F or until piping hot. Sprinkle with chopped coriander and serve.

The level of spice in this chilli dish is entirely up to you. Add more or less depending on your own taste.

Skinny HALOGEN OVEN
SIDE DISHES

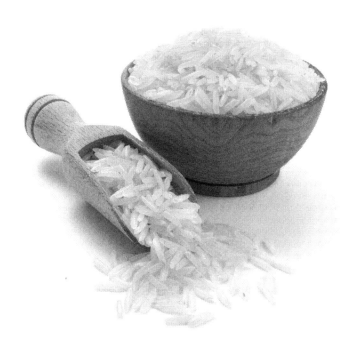

Baked Potato
Serves 1

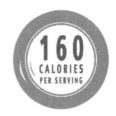

160 CALORIES PER SERVING

Ingredients:

Low-cal cooking oil spray
½ tsp crushed sea salt
125g/4oz Desiree potato
Salt & pepper to taste

Method:

Spray the potato with a little low-cal oil, pierce with a fork and use your hands to rub in the oil and crushed salt. Place in an ovenproof dish on the lower rack and leave to cook in the halogen oven at 200C/400F for 50-60 minutes or until tender. Cut in half, season well and serve.

Serve as a side dish to a meal or stuff with your favourite filling. Good low fat options include cottage cheese, tuna & capers and baked beans.

Garlic Baked Sweet Potato
Serves 1

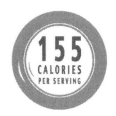

Ingredients:

Low-cal cooking oil spray
½ tsp crushed sea salt
150g/5oz sweet potato
2 garlic cloves, unpeeled
Salt & pepper to taste

Method:

Spray the potato and garlic cloves with a little low-cal oil, pierce the potato with a fork and use your hands to rub the oil and crushed salt into the skin. Place in an ovenproof dish on the lower rack and leave to cook in the halogen oven at 200C/400F for 50-60 minutes or until tender. Cut the potato in half and scoop out the flesh. Squeeze the garlic out of their skin and mash with a fork. Mix the garlic and soft potato flesh together, season and serve.

You can also serve as a traditional baked potato, rather than a mash, by loading the mixed garlic and potato flesh back into the empty skins.

Cauliflower Cream Cheese
Serves 1

140 CALORIES PER SERVING

Ingredients:

½ head large cauliflower, broken into florets
½ onion, chopped
1 tbsp breadcrumbs

1 tbsp low fat cream cheese
2 tbsp milk
Salt & pepper to taste

Method:

Steam the cauliflower florets until tender. Meanwhile gently heat together the cream cheese, onions and milk. Place the cauliflower in an ovenproof dish and pour over the cream cheese sauce. Season well and sprinkle on breadcrumbs. Place on the lower rack and leave to cook in the halogen oven at 240C/475F for 5-10 minutes or until golden brown.

Alter the recipe to include broccoli florets as well as cauliflower if you like. A tablespoon of tomato puree/ paste stirred through the cream cheese sauce is also good.

Tumeric Rice
Serves 1

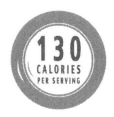

130
CALORIES
PER SERVING

Ingredients:

Low-cal cooking oil spray
60g/2 ½oz basmati rice
180ml/¾ cup vegetable stock
½ onion, chopped

1 bay leaf
1 tsp turmeric
Salt & pepper to taste

Method:

Gently sauté the onion in a little low-cal cooking oil. Add all
the ingredients to the pan and bring to the boil. Transfer to an
ovenproof dish and cover. Place on the lower rack and leave to
cook in the halogen oven at 200C/400F for 20-25 minutes or until
the rice is tender. Add a little more stock if needed. Remove the
bay leaf, drain, season and serve.

*The turmeric in this side dish gives the rice a really
strong yellow colour and a lovely aromatic smell.*

Grilled Tomatoes & Aubergines
Serves 1

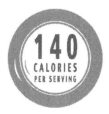

140 CALORIES PER SERVING

Ingredients:

Low-cal cooking oil spray
1 small aubergine/eggplant, thinly sliced
100g/3½oz tomatoes, thinly sliced

1 clove garlic, crushed
1 tbsp freshly chopped sage
Salt & pepper to taste

Method:

Lay the tomatoes and aubergine in a single layer in an ovenproof dish and spray with a little low-cal cooking oil. Brush with the crushed garlic, season and place on the upper rack of the halogen oven. Cook for 10-15 minutes at 240C/475F or until browned and tender.

This is a great side dish which you can serve with fish or meat. Alternatively double the quantities, sprinkle with parmesan cheese and serve as a main course.

Herbed Wedges
Serves 1

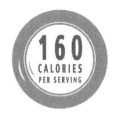

160 CALORIES PER SERVING

Ingredients:

Low-cal cooking oil spray
½ tsp crushed sea salt
125g/4oz Desiree potato
1 garlic clove, crushed

1 tbsp freshly chopped mixed herbs
Salt & pepper to taste

Method:

Leave the potato unpeeled and cut into wedges. Spray with a little low-cal oil and combine the salt, garlic and herbs well with the potato wedges. Place on a baking tray on the lower rack and leave to cook in the halogen oven at 220C/450F for 20-30 minutes or until golden & tender.

Desiree potatoes are ideal for this recipe but any potato should do well. Try basil and rosemary as the chopped herbs and also a pinch of chilli flakes if you like.

Rosemary & Garlic Mushrooms
Serves 1

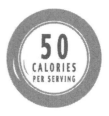

Ingredients:

Low-cal cooking oil spray
125g/4oz chestnut mushrooms,
sliced
2 garlic cloves, crushed

2 tbsp freshly chopped
rosemary
Salt and pepper to taste

Method:

Place all the ingredients in an ovenproof dish. Season well, place
on the high rack of the halogen oven and cook at 240C/475F for
6-8 minutes or until tender.

*If you are not too worried about calories, you could
use melted butter on the mushrooms rather than low-
cal cooking oil spray.*

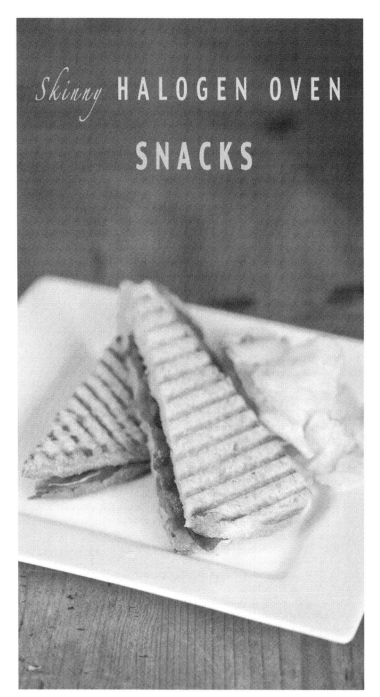

Skinny **HALOGEN OVEN**

SNACKS

Cheese On Toast
Serves 1

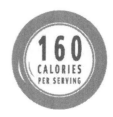

160 CALORIES PER SERVING

Ingredients:

1 slice wholegrain bread
25g/1oz gruyere cheese, grated
2 tsp worcestershire sauce
Salt & pepper to taste

Method:

Mix together the grated cheese and worcestershire sauce. Spread over the bread. Season and place on the grill pan/high rack of the halogen oven. Cook at 240C/475F for 4-5 minutes or until brown and bubbling.

If you are a marmite fan you can swap the worcestershire sauce by thinly spreading marmite over the bread before adding the cheese.

Mozzarella Ciabatta
Serves 1

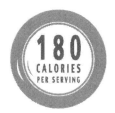

180 CALORIES PER SERVING

Ingredients:

Low-cal cooking oil spray
1 slice ciabatta bread
25g/1oz mozzarella cheese, chopped
2 cherry tomatoes, sliced

1 tsp tomato puree/paste
1 tsp basil leaves, chopped
Salt & pepper to taste

Method:

Spread the puree on the ciabatta bread. Lay the cheese and sliced cherry tomatoes on the bread. Season, spray with a little oil and place on the grill pan/high rack of the halogen oven. Cook at 240C/475F for 4-5 minutes or until the cheese is melted. Sprinkle with basil leaves and serve.

This is a simple and quick 'open' sandwich which is also good with sundried tomato paste.

Croque Monsieur Panini
Serves 1

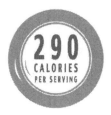

Ingredients:

1 panini sliced
1 slice emmental cheese
1 slice lean cured ham
Salt & pepper to taste

Method:

Place the cheese and ham inside the panini. Season and place on the grill pan/high rack of the halogen oven. Cook at 240C/475F for 4-5 minutes or until brown and bubbling. Turn once during cooking.

You can use any filling you prefer for you panini There are endless possibilities and your halogen oven will cook them super quick.

Rarebit Muffin
Serves 1

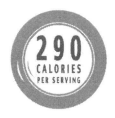

290 CALORIES PER SERVING

Ingredients:

1 breakfast muffin, split in two halves
1 tsp plain/all-purpose flour
3 tbsp milk

1 free range egg
25g/1oz mature cheddar, grated,
1 tsp Dijon mustard

Method:

Heat the milk in a pan and whisk in the flour. Take off the heat and mix in the cheese, egg and mustard. Pile on top of the breakfast muffins. Season and place on the grill pan/high rack of the halogen oven. Cook at 240C/475F for 4-5 minutes or until brown and bubbling.

For a stronger taste use English mustard rather than Dijon mustard.

Skinny HALOGEN OVEN
DESSERTS

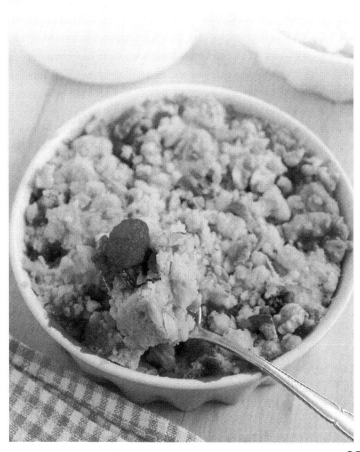

Sweet Lemon Bananas With Yoghurt
Serves 1

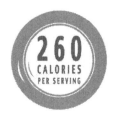

Ingredients:

2 ripe medium bananas, sliced
1 tbsp lemon juice
1 tbsp orange juice

2 tsp muscovado sugar
2 tbsp fat free Greek yoghurt
Pinch ground cinnamon

Method:

Mix together the sugar and juices. Place the bananas in an ovenproof dish and brush all over with the sugar and juice. Cover, place on the lower rack and leave to cook in the halogen oven for 10-15 minutes at 220C/450F. Serve with the Greek yoghurt on top sprinkled with ground cinnamon.

You could also serve this with ice cream or a flavoured yoghurt if you preferred, although watch out as this will alter the calorie count.

Pear Pudding
Serves 1

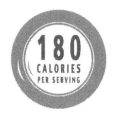

180 CALORIES PER SERVING

Ingredients:

2 small ripe pears, peeled,
cored and halved
1 tsp runny honey

1 tbsp orange juice
2 tbsp fat free Greek yoghurt
Pinch ground nutmeg

Method:

Mix together the honey and orange juice. Place the pear halves
in an ovenproof dish and brush all over with the honey and juice.
Cover, place on the lower rack and leave to cook in the halogen
oven for 20-25 minutes at 180C/350F or until the pears are tender.
Serve with Greek yoghurt on the side sprinkled with ground
nutmeg.

*It's best to peel the pears but if they are nice and ripe
don't worry too much if that's too fiddly.*

Spiced Sweet Apple & Prunes
Serves 1

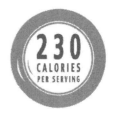

230 CALORIES PER SERVING

Ingredients:

1 large cooking apple, cored (not peeled)
1 tsp brown sugar
1 tbsp warm water
½ tsp each ground nutmeg & cinnamon

1 tsp runny honey
1 tbsp crème fraiche
2 dried prunes, chopped

Method:

Mix together the honey, sugar, water, prunes and spices. Stuff the cored apple, place in an ovenproof dish and pour any juices over the top. Cover, place on the lower rack and leave to cook in the halogen oven for 20-30 minutes at 200C/400F or until the apple is tender. Serve with crème fraiche dolloped on top of the apple.

The apple should be tender but not overcooked to the point of losing it's shape. Add more spices if you want a really aromatic pudding.

Soft Fruit Crumble
Serves 1

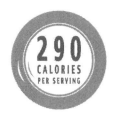

290 CALORIES PER SERVING

Ingredients:

150g/5oz blackberries, strawberries or ripe raspberries
2 tsp sugar
1 tbsp water
2 tsp golden syrup

2 tsp water
50g/2oz oats
2 tsp low fat 'butter' spread, melted

Method:

Mix together the sugar, water and soft fruit. Place in a small ovenproof dish and pour any juices over the top. Place on the lower rack and leave to cook in the halogen oven for 8-10 minutes at 200C/400F. Meanwhile mix together the syrup, oats & melted butter and place on top of the cooking soft fruit. Return to the oven and leave to cook for a further 14-18 minutes.

You may need to adjust the temperature for this pudding to make sure the crumble on top doesn't burn. Lovely served with fresh ice cream or just a dash of milk.

Vanilla Peaches
Serves 1

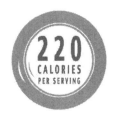

220 CALORIES PER SERVING

Ingredients:

200g/7oz sliced peaches,
tinned or fresh
1 tsp brown sugar

½ tsp vanilla extract
120ml/½ cup fat-free Greek
yoghurt

Method:

Mix together the sugar, vanilla extract and peach slices. Place in a small ovenproof dish on the lower rack of the halogen oven for 8-10 minutes at 200C/400F. Gently stir through the yoghurt and serve immediately.

If you use tinned peaches choose the type in its own juices rather than syrup. Also consider slightly lengthening the cooking time if you are using fresh peaches to make sure they are properly tender.

CONVERSION CHART: DRY INGREDIENTS

Metric	Imperial
7g	¼ oz
15g	½ oz
20g	¾ oz
25g	1 oz
40g	1½oz
50g	2oz
60g	2½oz
75g	3oz
100g	3½oz
125g	4oz
140g	4½oz
150g	5oz
165g	5½oz
175g	6oz
200g	7oz
225g	8oz
250g	9oz
275g	10oz
300g	11oz
350g	12oz
375g	13oz
400g	14oz

Metric	Imperial
425g	15oz
450g	1lb
500g	1lb 2oz
550g	1¼lb
600g	1lb 5oz
650g	1lb 7oz
675g	1½lb
700g	1lb 9oz
750g	1lb 11oz
800g	1¾lb
900g	2lb
1kg	2¼lb
1.1kg	2½lb
1.25kg	2¾lb
1.35kg	3lb
1.5kg	3lb 6oz
1.8kg	4lb
2kg	4½lb
2.25kg	5lb
2.5kg	5½lb
2.75kg	6lb

CONVERSION CHART: LIQUID MEASURES

Metric	Imperial	US
25ml	1fl oz	
60ml	2fl oz	¼ cup
75ml	2½ fl oz	
100ml	3½fl oz	
120ml	4fl oz	½ cup
150ml	5fl oz	
175ml	6fl oz	
200ml	7fl oz	
250ml	8½ fl oz	1 cup
300ml	10½ fl oz	
360ml	12½ fl oz	
400ml	14fl oz	
450ml	15½ fl oz	
600ml	1 pint	
750ml	1¼ pint	3 cups
1 litre	1½ pints	4 cups

Calorie Conscious

There is endless calorie information available for free online. It's almost impossible to put together a comprehensive resource as part of a book and so the list below is intended as nothing more than a guide to some of the more popular fruit, salad and vegetables to help you get a handle on food calories. All food calories are listed per 100g of the stated food.

Vegetables & Salad

Asparagus	20 cals
Benasprouts	30 cals
Broccoli	34 cals
Brussel Sprouts	42 cals
Butternut Squash	45 cals
Carotts	41 cals
Cauliflower	25 cals
Celery	14 cals
Courgette/Zucchini	16 cals
Cucumber	15 cals
Frozen Peas	64 cals
Green Peas	81 cals
Green Pepper	20 cals
Leeks	61 cals
Mixed Salad	17 cals
Mushrooms	22 cals
Pak Choi	13 cals
Parsnips	67 cals
Potatoes	75 cals
Red Cabbage	31 cals
Savoy Cabbage	27 cals
Spinach	23 cals
Sweet Potato	86 cals
Sweetcorn	86 cals
Tomatoes	18 cals
Wild Rocket	17 cals

Fruit

Appleds	52 cals
Avacado	160 cals
Banana	89 cals
Blackberries	43 cals
Blueberries	57 cals
Cantaloupe Melon	34 cals
Cherries	63 cals
Grapefruit	32 cals
Grapes	69 cals
Kiwi	61 cals
Oranges	47 cals
Peaches (canned)	44 cals
Peaches	39 cals
Pears	58 cals
Pineapple	48 cals
Plums	46 cals
Raspeberries	52 cals
Strawberries	32 cals
Watermelon	30 cals

Other
COOKNATION
TITLES

If you enjoyed 'The Skinny Halogen Oven Cooking For One Recipe Book' we'd really appreciate your feedback. Reviews help others decide if this is the right book for them so a moment of your time would be appreciated.

Thank you.

You may also be interested in other '**Skinny**' titles in the CookNation series. You can find all the following great titles by searching under '**CookNation**'.

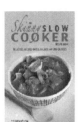

The Skinny Slow Cooker Recipe Book

Delicious Recipes Under 300, 400 And 500 Calories.

Paperback / eBook

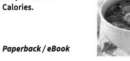

More Skinny Slow Cooker Recipes

75 More Delicious Recipes Under 300, 400 & 500 Calories.

Paperback / eBook

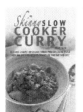

The Skinny Slow Cooker Curry Recipe Book

Low Calorie Curries From Around The World

Paperback / eBook

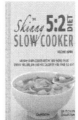
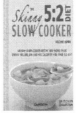

The Skinny Slow Cooker Soup Recipe Book

Simple, Healthy & Delicious Low Calorie Soup Recipes For Your Slow Cooker. All Under 100, 200 & 300 Calories.

Paperback / eBook

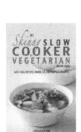

The Skinny Slow Cooker Vegetarian Recipe Book

40 Delicious Recipes Under 200, 300 And 400 Calories.

Paperback / eBook

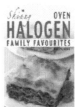

The Skinny 5:2 Slow Cooker Recipe Book

Skinny Slow Cooker Recipe And Menu Ideas Under 100, 200, 300 & 400 Calories For Your 5:2 Diet.

Paperback / eBook

The Skinny 5:2 Curry Recipe Book

Spice Up Your Fast Days With Simple Low Calorie Curries, Snacks, Soups, Salads & Sides Under 200, 300 & 400 Calories

Paperback / eBook

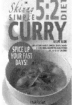

The Skinny Halogen Oven Family Favourites Recipe Book

Healthy, Low Calorie Family Meal-Time Halogen Oven Recipes Under 300, 400 and 500 Calories

Paperback / eBook

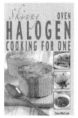

Skinny Halogen Oven Cooking For One

Single Serving, Healthy, Low Calorie Halogen Oven Recipes Under 200, 300 and 400 Calories

Paperback / eBook

Skinny Winter Warmers Recipe Book

Soups, Stews, Casseroles & One Pot Meals Under 300, 400 & 500 Calories.

Paperback / eBook

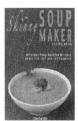

The Skinny Soup Maker Recipe Book

Delicious Low Calorie, Healthy and Simple Soup Recipes Under 100, 200 and 300 Calories. Perfect For Any Diet and Weight Loss Plan.

Paperback / eBook

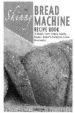

The Skinny Bread Machine Recipe Book

70 Simple, Lower Calorie, Healthy Breads...Baked To Perfection In Your Bread Maker.

Paperback / eBook

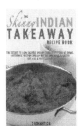

The Skinny Indian Takeaway Recipe Book

Authentic British Indian Restaurant Dishes Under 300, 400 And 500 Calories. The Secret To Low Calorie Indian Takeaway Food At Home

Paperback / eBook

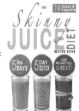

The Skinny Juice Diet Recipe Book

5lbs, 5 Days. The Ultimate Kick-Start Diet and Detox Plan to Lose Weight & Feel Great!

Paperback / eBook

The Skinny 5:2 Diet Recipe Book Collection

All The 5:2 Fast Diet Recipes You'll Ever Need. All Under 100, 200, 300, 400 And 500 Calories

Available only on eBook

eBook

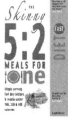

The Skinny 5:2 Fast Diet Meals For One

Single Serving Fast Day Recipes & Snacks Under 100, 200 & 300 Calories

Paperback / eBook

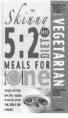

The Skinny 5:2 Fast Diet Vegetarian Meals For One

Single Serving Fast Day Recipes & Snacks Under 100, 200 & 300 Calories

Paperback / eBook

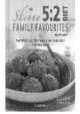

The Skinny 5:2 Fast Diet Family Favourites Recipe Book

Eat With All The Family On Your Diet Fasting Days

Paperback / eBook

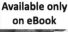

The Skinny 5:2 Fast Diet Family Favorites Recipe Book *U.S.A. EDITION*

Dine With All The Family On Your Diet Fasting Days

Available only on eBook

Paperback / eBook

The Skinny 5:2 Diet Chicken Dishes Recipe Book

Delicious Low Calorie Chicken Dishes Under 300, 400 & 500 Calories

Paperback / eBook

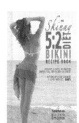

The Skinny 5:2 Bikini Diet Recipe Book

Recipes & Meal Planners Under 100, 200 & 300 Calories. Get Ready For Summer & Lose Weight...FAST!

Paperback / eBook

The Paleo Diet For Beginners Slow Cooker Recipe Book

Gluten Free, Everyday Essential Slow Cooker Paleo Recipes For Beginners

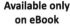

Available only on eBook

 eBook

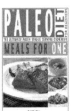

The Paleo Diet For Beginners Meals For One

The Ultimate Paleo Single Serving Cookbook

Paperback / eBook

The Paleo Diet For Beginners Holidays

Thanksgiving, Christmas & New Year Paleo Friendly Recipes

Available only on eBook *eBook*

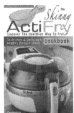

Available only on eBook

The Healthy Kids Smoothie Book

40 Delicious Goodness In A Glass Recipes for Happy Kids.

eBook

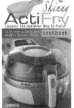

The Skinny Slow Cooker Summer Recipe Book

Fresh & Seasonal Summer Recipes For Your Slow Cooker. All Under 300, 400 And 500 Calories.

Paperback / eBook

The Skinny ActiFry Cookbook

Guilt-free and Delicious ActiFry Recipe Ideas: Discover The Healthier Way to Fry!

Paperback / eBook

The Skinny 15 Minute Meals Recipe Book

Delicious, Nutritious & Super-Fast Meals in 15 Minutes Or Less. All Under 300, 400 & 500 Calories.

Paperback / eBook

The Skinny Mediterranean Recipe Book

Simple, Healthy & Delicious Low Calorie Mediterranean Diet Dishes. All Under 200, 300 & 400 Calories.

Paperback / eBook

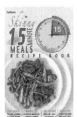
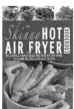

The Skinny Hot Air Fryer Cookbook

Delicious & Simple Meals For Your Hot Air Fryer: Discover The Healthier Way To Fry.

Paperback / eBook

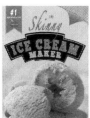

The Skinny Ice Cream Maker

Delicious Lower Fat, Lower Calorie Ice Cream, Frozen Yogurt & Sorbet Recipes For Your Ice Cream Maker

Paperback / eBook

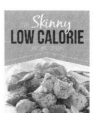

The Skinny Low Calorie Recipe Book

Great Tasting, Simple & Healthy Meals Under 300, 400 & 500 Calories. Perfect For Any Calorie Controlled Diet.

Paperback / eBook

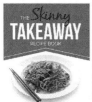

The Skinny Takeaway Recipe Book

Healthier Versions Of Your Fast Food Favourites: Chinese, Indian, Pizza, Burgers, Southern Style Chicken, Mexican & More. All Under 300, 400 & 500 Calories

Paperback / eBook

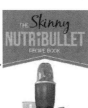

The Skinny Nutribullet Recipe Book

80+ Delicious & Nutritious Healthy Smoothie Recipes. Burn Fat, Lose Weight and Feel Great!

Paperback / eBook

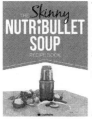

The Skinny Nutribullet Soup Recipe Book

Delicious, Quick & Easy, Single Serving Soups & Pasta Sauces For Your Nutribullet. All Under 100, 200, 300 & 400 Calories.

Paperback / eBook

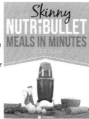

The Skinny Nutribullet Meals In Minutes Recipe Book

Quick & Easy, Single Serving Suppers, Snacks, Sauces, Salad Dressings & More. All Under 300, 400 & 500 Calories.

Paperback / eBook

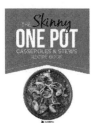

The Skinny One-Pot Recipe book

Simple & Delicious, One-Pot Meals. All Under 300, 400 & 500 Calories

Paperback / eBook

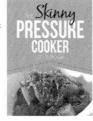

The Skinny Pressure Cooker Cookbook

USA ONLY

Low Calorie, Healthy & Delicious Meals, Sides & Desserts. All Under 300, 400 & 500 Calories.

Paperback / eBook

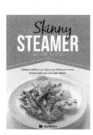

The Skinny Steamer Recipe Book

Delicious, Healthy, Low Calorie, Low Fat Steam Cooking Recipes Under 300, 400 & 500 Calories

Paperback / eBook

Printed in Great Britain
by Amazon